Veterinary Surgical Instruments: An Illustrated Guide

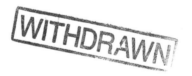

THE COLLEGE OF ANIMAL WELFARE

P.O. Box 165, Huntingdon

Veterinary Surgical Instruments: An Illustrated Guide

The College of Animal Welfare

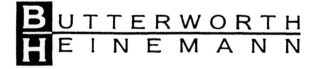

BUTTERWORTH-HEINEMANN
An imprint of Elsevier Limited

First published 1997
  Reprinted 2005, 2006

ISBN 0 7506 3613 0

British Library Cataloguing in Publication Data
A catalogue record for this book is available from the British Library

Library of Congress Cataloging in Publication Data
A catalog record for this book is available from the Library of Congress

Notice
Medical knowledge is constantly changing. Standard safety precautions must be
followed, but as new research and clinical experience broaden our knowledge,
changes in treatment and drug therapy may become necessary or appropriate.
Readers are advised to check the most current product information provided by
the manufacturer of each drug to be administered to verify the recommended dose,
the method and duration of administration, and contraindications. It is the
responsibility of the practitioner, relying on experience and knowledge of the
patient, to determine dosages and the best treatment for each individual patient.
Neither the Publisher nor the editors/contributor assumes any liability for any
injury and/or damage to persons or property arising from this publication.

The Publisher

ELSEVIER   your source for books,
           journals and multimedia
           in the health sciences
www.elsevierhealth.com

Working together to grow
libraries in developing countries

www.elsevier.com | www.bookaid.org | www.sabre.org

ELSEVIER   BOOK AID   Sabre Foundation
           International

The
Publisher's
policy is to use
**paper manufactured
from sustainable forests**

Typesetting and design by Coloursense Ltd., 95 Ashfield Street,
London E1

Transferred to digital printing 2006

Contents

GENERAL INSTRUMENTS   1

Artery Forceps   3
    Kocher Rochester Oschner   4
    Spencer Wells   4
    Halstead Mosquito   4

Scissors   7
    Mayo   8
    Metzenbaum   8
    Spencer Stitch   8
    Carless   10
    Standard   10
    Lister   10

Dissecting Forceps   13
    Standard, Plain and Toothed   14
    Continental Standard (End Toothed) 14
    Adsons   14
    Emmett   16
    Debakey   16

Tissue Forceps   19
    Allis   20
    Babcock   20
    Duval   20

Visceral Clamps   23
    Doyen Mayo-Robson   24
    Parker-Kerr   24

Towel Clamps   27
    Cross Action   28
    Backhaus   28

Scalpel Handles and Blades   31
    Scalpel Handles   32
    Scalpel Blades   32

Retractors - Handheld   35
    Langenbeck   36
    Hohmann   36
    Volkmann   36
    Czerny   38

Retractors - Self Retaining   41
    Gelpi   42
    Travers   42
    Cone   42
    Gosset   44
    Balfour   44
    Finochietto   44

Needle Holders   47
    Gillies   48
    Mayo Hegar   48
    Bruce Clarke   48
    Olsen Hegar   50
    McPhail   50

Diathermy Equipment   53
    Lead/Cable   54
    Quiver   54
    Beare Dissecting Forceps   56
    Robin Anchoring Clip   56

SPECIALIST EQUIPMENT   59

Orthopaedic Equipment   61
    Stille Chisel   62
    Stille Osteotome   62
    Stille Gouge   62
    Adson Periosteal Elevator   64
    Small Mallet   64
    Stille Luer Rongeurs   64
    Pennybacker Rongeurs   66
    Lempert Rongeurs   66
    Laminectomy Rongeurs   66
    Paton Bone Cutting Forceps   68
    Ruskin Liston Bone Cutting Forceps 68
    Fergusson Bone Cutting Forceps   68
    Hey Grove Bone Holding Forceps   70
    Kern Bone Holding Forceps and Cutters 70
    Jacobs Chuck for Intramedullary Pinning 70
    Wire Twisters   72
    Graft Passer   72
    Volkmann Curette   72

Implants   75
    Steinmann Pin   76
    Rush Pin   76
    Venables Plate   76

Sherman Plate 78
Dynamic Compression Plate 78
Reconstruction Plate 78
Cancellous Screw 80
Cortical Screw 80
Self Tapping Screw 80

ASIF Instruments **83**
Drill Bit 84
Drill Guide 84
Drill Sleeve 84
Depth Gauge 86
Tap 86
Tap Handle 86
Screwdriver 88
Countersink 88

Ophthalmic Instruments **91**
Iris Scissors 92
Tenotomy (Stevens) Scissors 92
Castroviejo Scissors 92
Catford Forceps 94
Chalazion Forceps 94
Bennett Cilia Forceps 94
Capsulorhexis Forceps 96
Micro Corneal Tying Forceps 96
Capsule Forceps 96
Kirby Expressor Hook and Lens Loop 98
Williams Speculum 98
Barraquer Speculum 98
Nettleship Dilator 100
Castroviejo Needle Holders 100

Dental Instruments **103**
Extraction Forceps 104
Dental Elevator 104
Periosteal Elevator 104
Subgingival Curette 106
Supragingival Scaler 106
Dental Explorer 108
Peridontal Probe 108
Sharpening Stone 108

Miscellaneous Instruments **111**
Cusco Vaginal Speculum 112
Hartmann Crocodile Forceps 112
Rampley Sponge Holding Forceps 112
Cheatle Sterilising Forceps 114

Acknowledgements

The college is most grateful for the help of Andrea Jeffery (VN DipAVN(Surgical)) in the preparation of this book.

The College would also like to thank the following companies for allowing the reproduction of their photographs:

Rocket Medical
Imperial Way
Watford
WD2 4XX

STRATEC Medical
20 Tewin Road
Welwyn Garden City
AL7 1LG

Veterinary Instrumentation
62 Cemetery Road
Sheffield
S11 9FP

John Weiss & Son Ltd
89 Alston Drive
Bradwell Abbey
Milton Keynes
MK13 9HF

...... and the following people for their advice and expertise during the writing of this book:

David Crossley BVetMed MRCVS F AVD
Christine Heinrich MRCVS Cert V Optical
Nick Jeffery Cert SAO DSAS BVSc FRCVS
Sally Turner MA VetMB DV Ophth MRCVS

Introduction

The aim of this book is to aid nurses and students to identify commonly used, widely available instruments. It has not been written to contain an exhaustive list of instruments (at present there are 378 designs of extraction forceps available in dentistry alone). It is very important to note that veterinary surgeons will always have personal preferences and uses for instruments.

Having studied this book it would be pleasing to think that the next time a veterinary surgeon says:

"Pass those things that have the funny shaped tips, you know, those double jointed things I always use. No, not those, the things next to them. Yeah! That's them!"

You can confidently reply:

"Do you mean the Stille Luer Rongeurs?"

General Instruments

Artery Forceps

Scissors

Dissecting Forceps

Tissue Forceps

Visceral Clamps

Towel Clamps

Scalpel Handles and Blades

Retractors - Handheld

Retractors - Self Retaining

Needle Holders

Diathermy Equipment

Artery Forceps

Common Features

Ratchet to maintain a closed position

Serrated blades

Clamp tightly shut

Ring grip for fingers

Screw or box joint

Use

Occlusion of blood vessels

Kocher Rochester Oschner

Name	Kocher Rochester Oschner (straight and curved)
Purpose	Clamping blood vessels
Size	13 - 20 cm
Distinguishing Features	Teeth at tips
Similar Instruments	Mayo Oschner

Spencer Wells

Name	Spencer Wells (straight and curved)
Purpose	Clamping blood vessels
Size	13 - 20 cm
Distinguishing Features	None
Similar Instruments	Mayo, Moynihan, Rochester

Halstead Mosquito

Name	Halstead Mosquito (straight and curved)
Purpose	Clamping small blood vessels
Size	12.5 cm
Distinguishing Features	Small, fine tipped artery forceps
Similar Instruments	Kelly

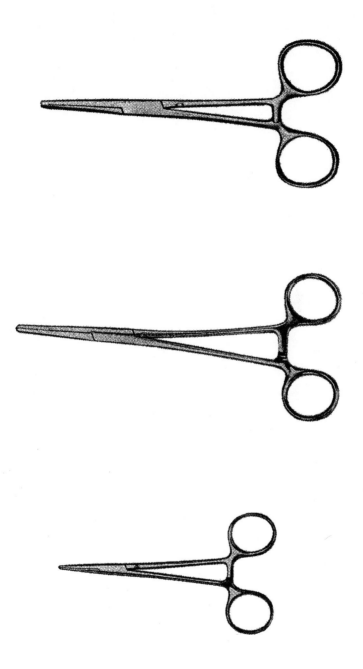

Scissors

Common Features

Two blades

Uses

Sharp and blunt soft tissue dissection (not skin)

Suture cutting

Mayo

Name	Mayo (straight and curved)
Purpose	Soft tissue dissection and cutting
Size	14 - 21.5 cm
Distinguishing Features	Smooth tips
Similar Instruments	Mayo-Stille, Aufrichts

Metzenbaum

Name	Metzenbaum
Purpose	Soft tissue dissection (fine)
Size	14 - 21.5 cm
Distinguishing Features	Long handle, short blade
Similar Instruments	Nelson, McIndoe

Spencer Stitch

Name	Spencer Stitch
Purpose	Suture removal
Size	9 - 13 cm
Distinguishing Features	Shape of tip specifically for suture removal
Similar Instruments	None

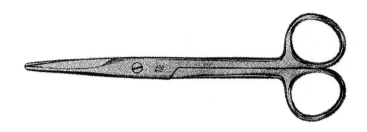

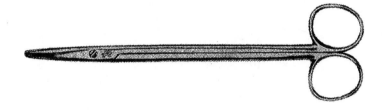

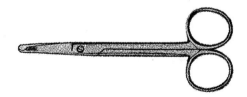

Carless

Name	Carless
Purpose	Suture cutting
Size	17 - 20 cm
Distinguishing Features	Square, blunt tips
Similar Instruments	Standard blunt/blunt

Standard

Name	Standard (straight and curved, sharp or blunt.
Purpose	Cutting fur or sutures
Size	10 - 20 cm
Distinguishing Features	Different shaped blades
Similar Instruments	Nurses scissors

Lister

Name	Lister
Purpose	Bandage cutting/removal
Size	14 - 20 cm
Distinguishing Features	Angled beyond joint with a flattened tip
Similar Instruments	Stadler

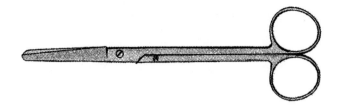

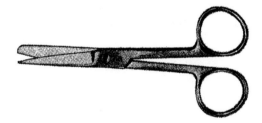

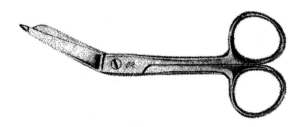

Dissecting Forceps

Common Features

Handle with serration for grip

Tips may be rat toothed or serrated

Use

Intermittent, temporary grasping of:

    tissue

    skin

    soft tissue

    viscera

Standard, Plain and Toothed

Name	Continental Standard
Purpose	Handling soft tissue
Size	11.5 - 30 cm
Distinguishing Features	Rounded serrated tips
Similar Instruments	Bonney (plain) Lane

Continental Standard (End Toothed)

Name	Continental Standard (End Toothed)
Purpose	Handling skin
Size	11.5 - 30 cm
Distinguishing Features	Narrow, rat toothed tips
Similar Instruments	Semkin, Gillies

Adsons

Name	Adsons (plain end)
Purpose	Fine handling of soft tissue
Size	13 - 18 cm
Distinguishing Features	Widened area proximal to the tips
Similar Instruments	Gillies, McIndoe

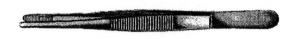

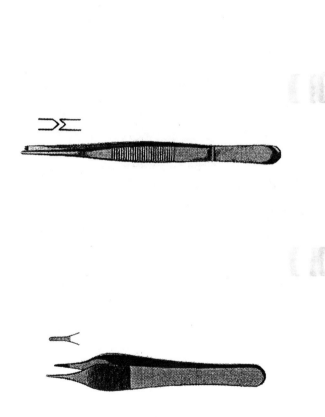

Emmett

Name	Emmett
Purpose	Handling deep, soft tissue (e.g., uterus)
Size	20 cm
Distinguishing Features	Long, thin tips with a broad proximal portion
Similar Instrument	None

Debakey

Name	Debakey
Purpose	Atraumatic handling of viscera Useful for abdominal and thoracic surgery
Size	15 cm, 18 cm, 19.5 cm
Distinguishing Features	Longitudinal grooves along both tips
Similar Instruments	Cooley Forceps

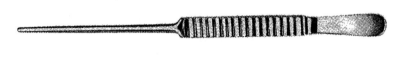

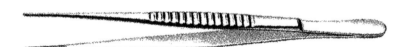

Tissue Forceps

Common Features

Ring grip for fingers

Ratchet maintains a closed position

Tip has a fine area of contact

Uses

Prolonged grasping of soft tissue or viscera

Allis

Name	Allis
Purpose	Handling soft tissue (not viscera)
Size	15cm, 20 cm
Distinguishing Features	Tip rounded with teeth on the gripping surface
Similar Instruments	Judd-Allis, Stiles

Babcock

Name	Babcock Intestinal Forceps
Purpose	Handling soft tissue and viscera
Size	15 - 23 cm
Distinguishing Features	Tip shape triangular and curved longitudinal lines on the grasping surface Finer ends than the Allis Tissue Forceps
Similar Instruments	Duval

Duval

Name	Duval
Purpose	Handling soft tissue and viscera (lung lobes)
Size	19 cm
Distinguishing Features	Flattened triangular tip Fine teeth along the gripping surface
Similar Instruments	Babcock

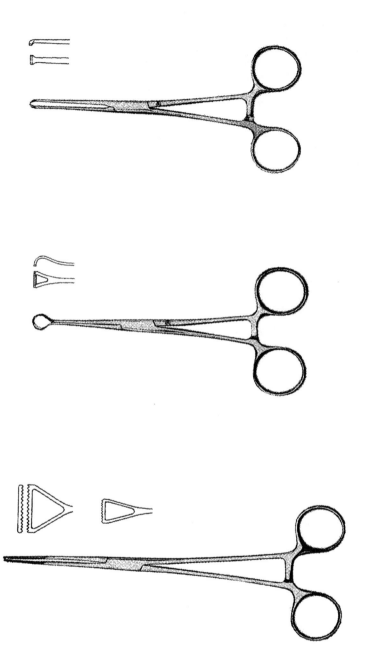

Visceral Clamps

Common Features

Ring grip for fingers

Ratchet maintains a closed position

Flattened, elongated clamps

Use

Occluding visceral lumen

Doyen Mayo-Robson

Name	Doyen Mayo-Robson
Purpose	Visceral occlusion (intestine and stomach)
Size	24 cm
Distinguishing Features	Gap between grasping surfaces
Similar Instruments	Lane

Parker-Kerr

Name	Parker-Kerr
Purpose	Occlusion of viscera, e.g., cervix
Size	25 cm
Distinguishing Features	Heavy forceps with curved tips and screw joint No gap between the grasping surfaces
Similar Instruments	Geary Grant Cholecystectomy Forceps

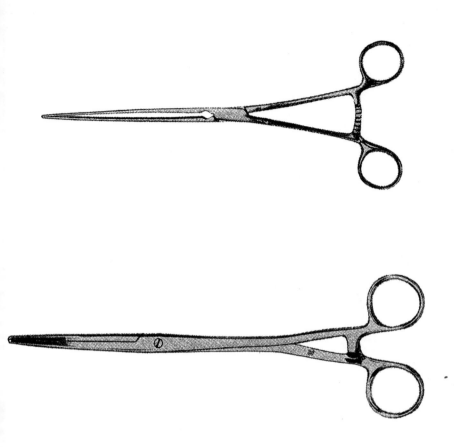

Towel Clamps

Common Features

Sharp curved tips which cross over

Use

Anchoring drapes to the patient

Cross Action

Name	Cross Action
Purpose	Anchoring drapes to the surgical field
Size	9.5 - 13.5 cm
Distinguishing Features	Spring type cross action
Similar Instruments	Jones, Schaedel

Backhaus

Name	Backhaus
Purpose	Anchoring drapes to the surgical field
Size	9.5 cm
Distinguishing Features	Box joint and ratchet
Similar Instruments	Duff (has teeth at tip and screw joint)

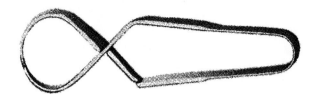

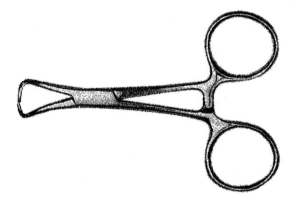

Scalpel Handles and Blades

Common Features

Diagonal ledge near tip

Central raised area on tip

Use

Holding scalpels

Scalpel Handles

Name   Scalpel Handles, Size No 3, 4 and 5

Purpose   For attachment of scalpel blades

Size   No 3, 4 and 5

Distinguishing Features   The No 5 handle is longer and narrow
                            None of them could be mistaken for anything else

Similar Instruments   None

Scalpel Blades

Name   Scalpel Blades, Size Nos 10, 11, 12, 15 and 20

Purpose   Tissue incision and transection

Size   Nos 10, 11, 12, 15 and 20

Distinguishing Features   See illustrations

Similar Instruments   None

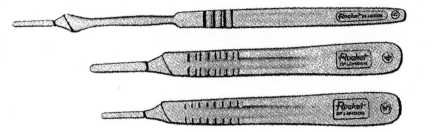

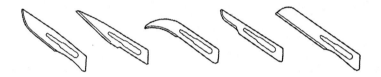

Retractors - Handheld

Common Features

Grooved handle

Hook-like end - may be flattened

Uses

Retraction of soft tissue, viscera and bone

Langenbeck

Name	Langenbeck
Purpose	Soft tissue retraction to expose other structures
Size	23 x 7 mm, 44 x 13 mm, 64 x 26 mm
Distinguishing Features	Flat blade "L" shaped retractor Grooved handle
Similar Instruments	Morris

Hohmann

Name	Hohmann
Purpose	Retraction within a joint
Size	12 mm and 18 mm wide
Distinguishing Features	Small beak at the tip of the retractor
Similar Instruments	None

Volkmann

Name	Volkmann
Purpose	Retraction of tendon and muscle to expose other structures
Size	21.5 cm
Distinguishing Features	Tip looks like a rake
Similar Instruments	Senn

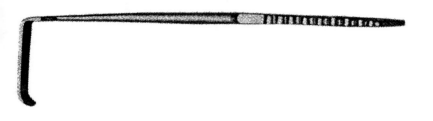

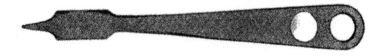

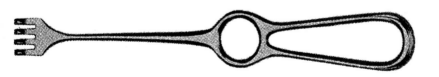

Czerny

Name	Czerny
Purpose	Soft tissue retraction
Size	18 cm
Distinguishing Features	Flat blade at one end and a double prong at the other
Similar Instruments	Mathieu

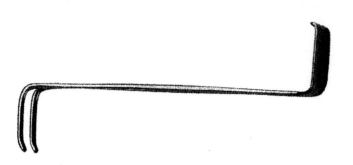

Retractors - Self Retaining

Common Features

Ratchet which maintains open position

Uses

Prolonged retraction of soft tissue, viscera and bone

41

Gelpi

Name	Gelpi (sharp or blunt)
Purpose	Muscle and joint retraction
Size	18 cm
Distinguishing Features	Single pronged outwardly turning tips
Similar Instruments	None

Travers

Name	Travers
Purpose	Muscle and joint retraction
Size	20 cm
Distinguishing Features	Four teeth on each side with blunt tips
Similar Instruments	West Weislander (smaller than Travers being 14 cm) Weislander (four teeth on one side and three teeth on the other - smaller than Travers being 14 cm)

Cone

Name	Cone
Purpose	Retraction of muscle during orthopaedic procedures
Size	25 cm
Distinguishing Features	Joints half way along the arms to allow a flexible field of retraction
Similar Instruments	Travers, West, Weislander (none of these have the joint along each arm)

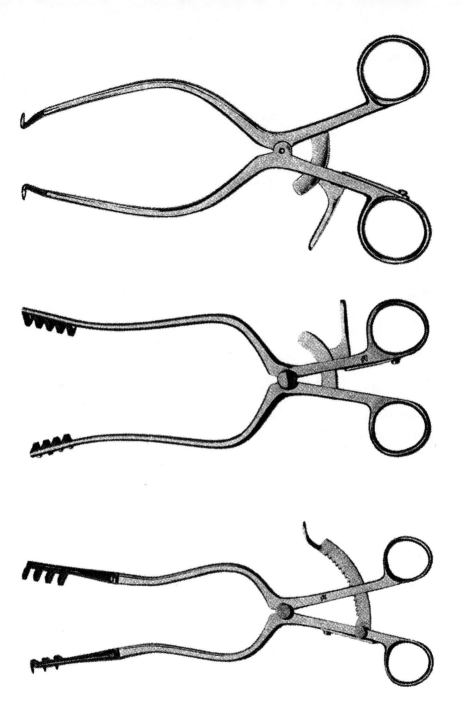

Gosset

Name	Gosset
Purpose	Abdominal wall retraction
Size	Adult and infant sizes
Distinguishing Features	Square shape with straight arms No central retraction blade
Similar Instruments	None

Balfour

Name	Balfour
Purpose	Abdominal wall and liver retraction
Size	Standard size
Distinguishing Features	Curved arms and a central refractor blade with a wingnut
Similar Instrument	Bourne

Finochietto

Name	Finochietto
Purpose	Rib spreaders
Size	Standard size
Distinguishing Features	Toothed bracket (comb like) for retractor blade attachment
Similar Instruments	Tuffier

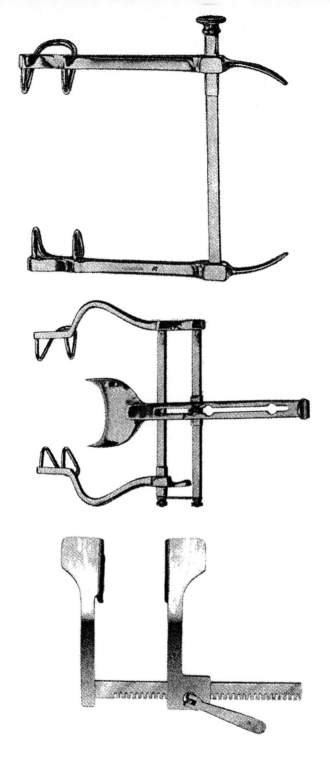

Needle Holders

Common Features

Flat tips of blades with stippled surface

Often have ring shaped finger grips

Often have ratchet to maintain closure

May be combined with scissor blades

Uses

Holding needles

Cutting sutures

Gillies

Name	Gillies (handheld)
Purpose	Holding needles and cutting sutures
Size	16 cm
Distinguishing Features	One handle shorter than the other with larger thumb/finger grip Has a cutting edge
Similar Instruments	None

Mayo Hegar

Name	Mayo Hegar (self retaining) (gold handles indicateTungsten Carbide tips)
Purpose	Holding needles
Size	14 - 20 cm
Distinguishing Features	Flat tips not serrated (as in artery forceps) Indentation on grasping surface (see picture) which similar instruments do not have
Similar Instruments	Wright

Bruce Clarke

Name	Bruce Clarke (self retaining)
Purpose	Holding needles
Size	13 cm
Distinguishing Features	When closed, small circular holes are apparent along the length of the grasping surface
Similar Instruments	None

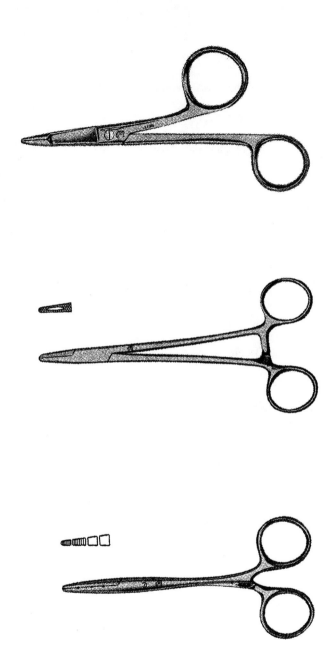

Olsen Hegar

Name	Olsen Hegar (self retaining)
Purpose	Holding needles and cutting sutures
Size	14 cm and 17 cm
Distinguishing Features	Scissors incorporated distal to the needle holding tips
Similar Instruments	None

McPhail

Name	McPhail (self retaining with copper lined jaw)
Purpose	Holding needles
Size	18 cm
Distinguishing Features	Copper lined jaws and pear shaped handles
Similar Instruments	None

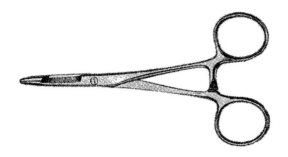

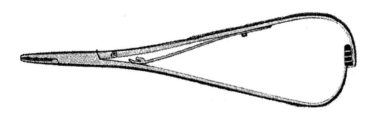

51

Diathermy Equipment

Lead/Cable

Name	Lead/cable (red rubber)
Purpose	For attachment of diathermy blade/forceps to the machine
Size	Standard length
Distinguishing Features	Hook at one end for attachment to the diathermy machine Usually made of red rubber
Similar Instruments	Bipolar diathermy cable

Quiver

Name	Quiver
Purpose	Holding diathermy blade/forceps/scissors
Size	Standard size
Distinguishing Features	Plastic hollow container with a ring at the top to secure with a towel clamp onto a drape
Similar Instruments	None

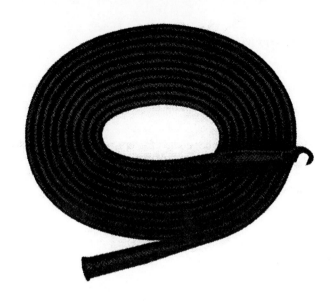

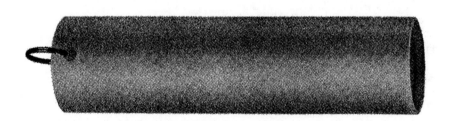

Beare Dissecting Forceps

Name	Beare Dissecting Forceps
Purpose	Holding tissues/vessels while diathermy takes place
Size	15 cm
Distinguishing Features	Rubber coated forceps (except tip and insertion) to connect to a diathermy lead
Similar Instruments	Waugh

Robin Anchoring Clip

Name	Robin Anchoring Clip
Purpose	Anchoring diathermy lead to drapes
Size	13 cm
Distinguishing Features	Bracket on either side of the body to hold diathermy lead
Similar Instruments	Could be confused with a Backhaus Towel Clamp

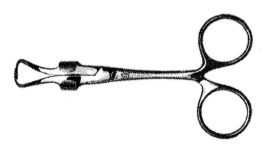

57

Specialist Equipment

Orthopaedic Equipment

Implants

ASIF Equipment (Association for the Study of Internal Fixation)

Ophthalmic Instruments

Dental Instruments

Miscellaneous Instruments

Orthopaedic Equipment

Chisel

Name	Stille Chisel
Purpose	To shave bone
Size	20 cm
Distinguishing Features	Bevelled on <u>one</u> side only to allow the instrument to sit flush with bone
Similar Instruments	Osteotome

Osteotome

Name	Stille Osteotome
Purpose	To make a precise bone cut (e.g., trochanteric osteotomy, excision arthroplasty)
Size	20 cm
Distinguishing Features	Tip bevelled on <u>both</u> sides
Similar Instruments	Chisel

Gouge

Name	Stille Gouge
Purpose	To shave bone where bone contouring is needed
Size	20 cm
Distinguishing Features	Crescent moon-shaped tip
Similar Instruments	Osteotome, Chisel, Periosteal Elevator

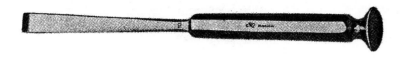

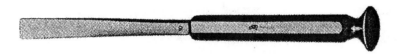

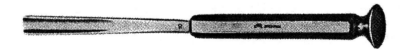

63

Periosteal Elevator

Name	Adson Periosteal Elevator
Purpose	Raise periosteum from bone before plating or drilling
Size	Jaw width 7 mm
Distinguishing Features	Rounded, curved tip
Similar Instruments	Bristow, Farabeuf

Mallet

Name	Small Mallet
Purpose	For use with chisels, gouges and osteotomes
Size	Weight 250 g (8.5 oz)
Distinguishing Features	It looks like a mallet
Similar Instruments	Heath

Rongeurs

Name	Stille Luer Rongeurs
Purpose	Nibbling pieces of bone
Size	21.5 cm
Distinguishing Features	Double action joint, small projections on handles Lever action to spring back into open position Cup like cutting tips
Similar Instruments	Jansen Middleton

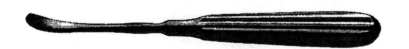

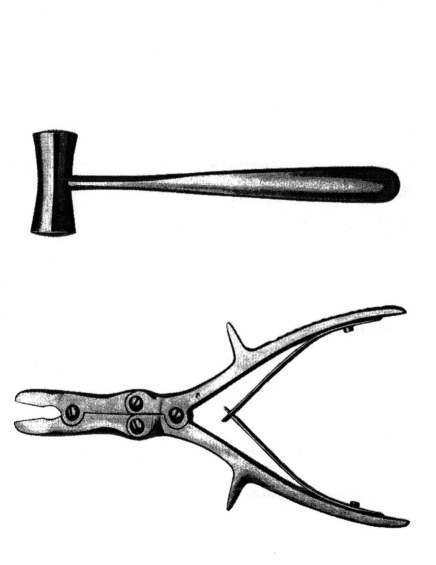

Rongeurs

Name	Pennybacker Rongeurs
Purpose	Nibbling pieces of bone
Size	20 cm
Distinguishing Features	Spring action handles Cup like cutting tips
Similar Instruments	Northfield

Rongeurs

Name	Lempert Rongeurs
Purpose	Removal (fine) of bone and soft tissue in neurosurgery
Size	19 cm
Distinguishing Features	Fine tips
Similar Instruments	Cicherelli

Rongeurs

Name	Laminectomy Rongeurs
Purpose	Removal of cortical bone during certain spinal surgery
Size	Jaw widths 2, 3 and 4 mm
Distinguishing Features	Handles angled to allow good vision of surgical site Slim lower jaw
Similar Instruments	None

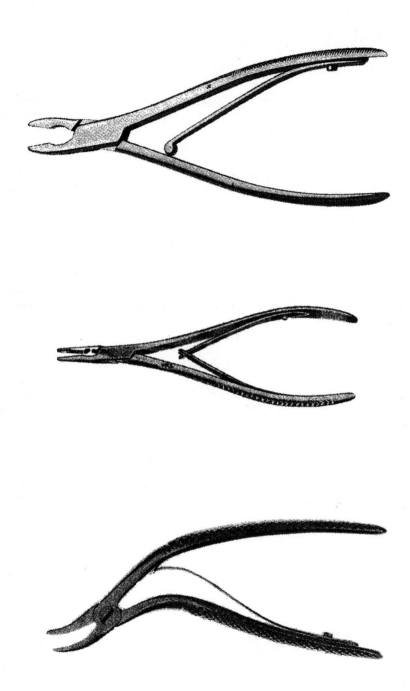

67

Bone Cutting Forceps

Name	Paton Bone Cutting Forceps
Purpose	To cut pieces of bone
Size	14 cm
Distinguishing Features	Single action bone cutting forceps Lever action in the centre Flat, sloping blades.
Similar Instruments	Liston

Bone Cutting Forceps

Name	Ruskin Liston (angled and straight) Bone Cutting Forceps
Purpose	To cut pieces of bone
Size	15 cm and 20 cm
Distinguishing Features	Double action joint allowing for less physical force to cut bone Delicate cutting blades
Similar Instruments	None

Bone Holding Forceps

Name	Fergusson Bone Holding Forceps
Purpose	Securing bone to prevent movement during orthopaedic procedures
Size	15 cm
Distinguishing Features	Heavy instrument Double toothed grip at the tip Not self retaining
Similar Instruments	None

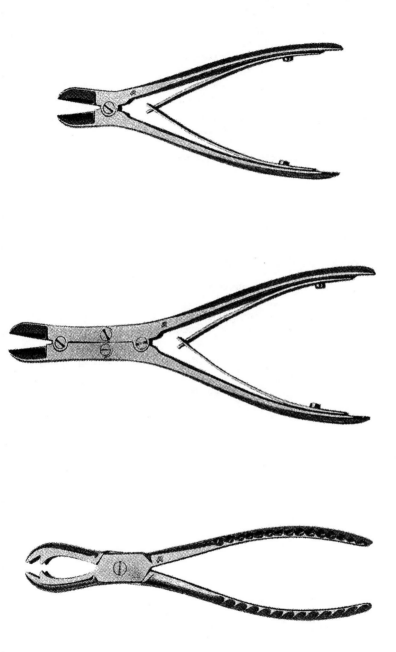

Bone Holding Forceps

Name	Hey Grove Bone Holding Forceps
Purpose	Securing bone to prevent movement during orthopaedic procedures
Size	20, 25 and 30 cm
Distinguishing Features	Wing nut maintains closure of the tips
Similar Instruments	None

Bone Holding Forceps

Name	Kern Bone Holding Forceps
Purpose	Securing bone to prevent movement during orthopaedic procedures
Size	15cm and 16 cm
Distinguishing Features	Four pointed prongs on jaws for a non-slip grip
Similar Instruments	Lane Bone Holding Forceps

Jacobs Chuck for Intramedullary Pinning

Name	Jacobs Chuck for intramedullary pinning
Purpose	Introduction or extraction of pins, e.g., K wires and Steinmann pins
Size	Small (4 mm capacity) Standard (6 mm capacity)
Distinguishing Features	A very heavy instrument It has a hole through the centre of it to allow pin to be held Has a key with it to close aperture of three teeth around pin
Similar Instruments	None

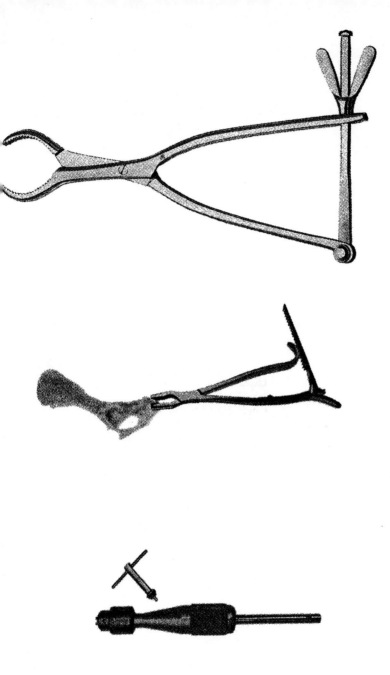

Wire Twisters and Cutters

Name	Wire Twisters and Cutters
Purpose	Securing cerclage and tension band wires after placement
Size	16 cm
Distinguishing Features	Serrated jaws Look like pliers
Similar Instruments	ASIF wire twisters

Graft Passer

Name	Graft Passer
Purpose	Surgery for cruciate deficient stifle joints
Size	Head size 2 cm, 3 cm, 4.5 cm and 6 cm
Distinguishing Features	Curved head with a hole at the tip, like a giant sewing needle with a handl.
Similar Instruments	Wire passer - this has a curved head with a hole running through the centre of it

Curette

Name	Volkmann Curette
Purpose	Scraping cavities, eg, bone grafts and debridement
Size	16 cm
Distinguishing Features	Double ended One end has a round cup and the other has an oval cup
Similar Instruments	House Curette, Spratt Curette

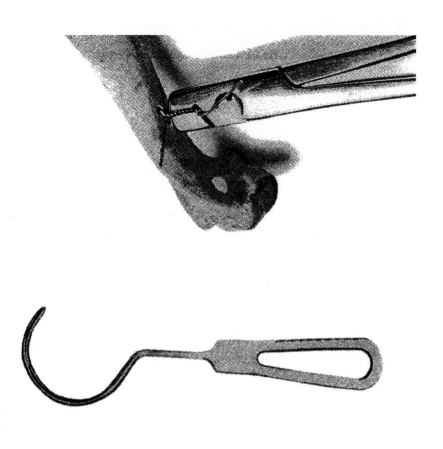

Implants

Pins

Name	Steinmann Pin (trochar, bevelled, screw tips)
Purpose	Orthopaedics
Size	Various diameters 1.6 - 8 mm
Distinguishing Features	The diameter of the pin indicate the pin type Kirschner pins have much smaller diameters
Similar Instruments	Kirschner wire/pin

Pins

Name	Rush Pin
Purpose	Used in pairs for repair of the proximal and distal third of long bones
Size	2.5 mm + 3 mm diameter (various lengths)
Distinguishing Features	Looks like a shepherd's crook at one end, flattened at the other end
Similar Instruments	None

Plates

Name	Venables Plate
Purpose	Fracture fixation
Size	Various lengths and numbers of holes
Distinguishing Features	Rectangular plate with round holes
Similar Instruments	Dynamic Compression Plate

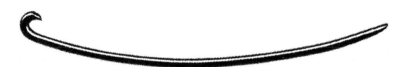

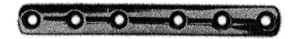

Plates

Name	Sherman Plate
Purpose	Fracture fixation
Size	Various lengths and numbers of holes
Distinguishing Features	The plate looks like the tracks on a sherman tank, ie, narrower between the holes
Similar Instruments	Burns and Lane

Plates

Name	Dynamic Compression Plate
Purpose	Fracture fixation and compression
Size	1.5 mm, 2.0 mm, 2.7 mm, 3.5 mm and 4.5 mm (narrow and broad)
Distinguishing Features	Rectangular plate with <u>oval</u> holes
Similar Instruments	Venables Plate

Plates

Name	Reconstruction Plate
Purpose	Fracture fixation and compression
Size	2 mm, 2.4 mm, 2.7 mm, 3.5 mm and 4.5 mm
Distinguishing Features	Rectangular plate with <u>oval</u> holes and bites taken out of each side
Similar Instruments	None

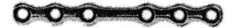

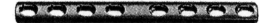

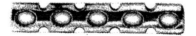

Screws

Name	Cancellous Screw (pre-tapped)
Purpose	For securing a plate to cancellous bone and re-attaching bone fragments
Size	3.5 mm, 4 mm and 6.5 mm
Distinguishing Features	Coarser thread than cortical screw for better "bite" into bone Blunt tip
Similar Instruments	Cortical Bone Screw

Screws

Name	Cortical Screw (pre-tapped)
Purpose	For securing a plate to cortical bone and re-attaching bone fragments
Size	2.0 mm, 2.7 mm, 3.5 mm and 4.5 mm
Distinguishing Features	Fine wedge shaped thread Hexagonal shaped hole in head Blunt tip
Similar Instruments	Cancellous Screws (pre-tapped)

Screws

Name	Self tapping Screw
Purpose	Plate fixation and re-attachment of bone fragments
Size	2.0 mm, 2.7 mm and 3.5 mm
Distinguishing Features	Sharp tip
Similar Instruments	Cancellous /cortical pre-tapped screws

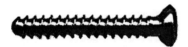

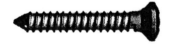

ASIF Equipment
Association for the Study of Internal Fixation

Drill Bit

Name	Drill Bit (quick coupling)
Purpose	To drill a hole into bone
Size	1.1 - 4.5 mm diameter
Distinguishing Features	Distal end tapered for quick coupling (as with tap)
Similar Instruments	Drill bit for other drills and Jacob Chuck

Drill Guide

Name	Drill Guide
Purpose	To guide and support the drill bit into the correct position during drilling through a plate in the neutral and load positions
Size	Must correspond with drill bit and plate sizes
Distinguishing Features	Long body with angled tips with coloured inserts at both ends
Similar Instruments	Other drill guides

Drill Sleeve

Name	Drill Sleeve
Purpose	To protect tissue from drill bits and taps
Size	Must correspond with the drill bit
Distinguishing Features	Long body with angled tips of uniform shape
Similar Instruments	Universal drill guide

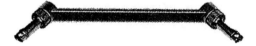

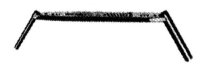

Depth Gauge

Name	Depth Gauge
Purpose	Measures the depth of the hole made in bone to enable exact length of screw to be selected
Size	One for 4.5 to 6.5 mm screws One for 2.7 to 4.0 mm screws One for 1.5 to 2.0 mm screws
Distinguishing Features	Narrow hooked tip and an adjustable ruler
Similar Instruments	None

Tap

Name	Tap for Cortical Bone Screws
Purpose	Cuts a thread into bone for the secure anchoring of non-self tapping screws
Size	Must correspond with screw size
Distinguishing Features	Distal end looks like the screw thread with vertical grooves cut into it. Quick coupling distal end (as with drill bit)
Similar Instruments	Tap for cancellous bone screws (thread is deeper)

Tap Handle

Name	Tap Handle (with quick couple)
Purpose	For attachment of the tap to enable use by the operator
Size	Corresponds with screw sizes
Distinguishing Features	The tap handle for the 2.7 mm, 3.5 mm and 4.5 mm cortical and 6.5 mm cancellous screws is T shaped
Similar Instruments	None

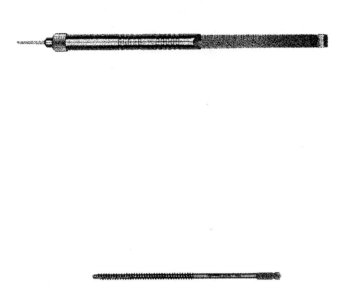

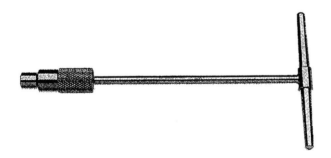

Screwdriver

Name	Screwdriver
Purpose	To screw screws into bone
Size	Corresponds with screw size
Distinguishing Features	All ASIF screwdrivers have a hexagonal head
Similar Instruments	None

Countersink (Quick Coupling)

Name	Countersink (quick coupling)
Purpose	To allow screws to sit flush with bone when a plate is not being used It also disperses forces from below the screw head.
Size	To correspond with screw size
Distinguishing Features	Fluted tip with nipple on end
Similar Instruments	None

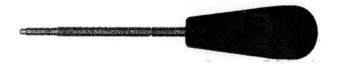

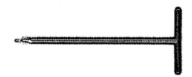

Ophthalmic Instruments

Scissors

Name	Iris Scissors
Purpose	Cutting the iris. General purpose conjunctival scissors
Size	12 mm cutting length
Distinguishing Features	Small sharp scissors
Similar Instruments	Williamson - Noble Iris Scissors

Scissors

Name	Tenotomy (Stevens)
Purpose	For fine dissection during intra-ocular surgery
Size	20 - 35 mm blade length
Distinguishing Features	A tapering shaped end
Similar Instruments	None

Scissors

Name	Castroviejo - Vannus Capsulotomy (straight and curved)
Purpose	To cut away the anterior lens capsule during cataract surgery
Size	6 mm cutting length
Distinguishing Features	Spring action pear shaped handle and tiny blades
Similar Instruments	None

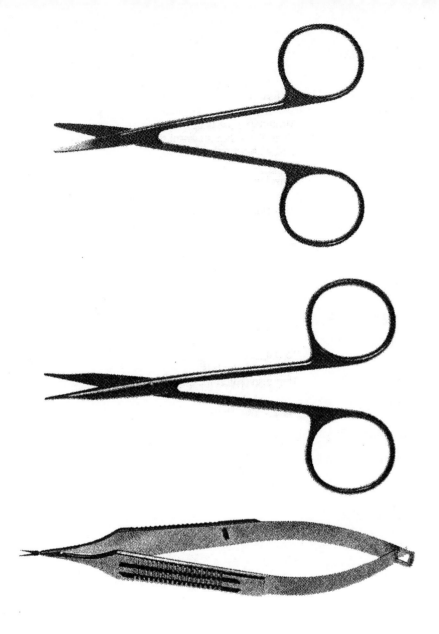

Forceps

Name	Catford Micro-corneal Forceps (with or without teeth)
Purpose	Atraumatic grasping of the cornea and sutures There is a tying platform which allows sutures to be held without risk of fraying
Size	9 cm long
Distinguishing Features	Very fine tips with a tying platform
Similar Instruments	Castroviejo, MacPherson and Harms Forceps

Forceps

Name	Chalazion Forceps
Purpose	To stabilise the eyelids and provide haemostasis during surgery on the lids They also protect the underlying globe during cryosurgery.
Size	Plate width 26 mm. Instrument length 8.5 cm..
Distinguishing Features	Oval tip with solid back plate
Similar Instruments	Tarsal Cyst Forceps, Wilde Entropian Forceps

Forceps

Name	Bennett Cilia Forceps
Purpose	For plucking distichia (extra eye lashes)
Size	6.5 mm long
Distinguishing Features	Small round tips with a hole in the centre
Similar Instruments	Round-end Cilia Forceps

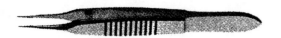

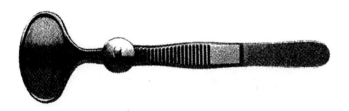

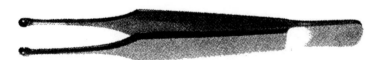

Forceps

Name	Capsulorhexis Forceps
Purpose	To grasp and tear the lens capsule
Size	11 cm (length)
Distinguishing Features	Very fine tips with hooked ends
Similar Instruments	None

Forceps

Name	Micro-corneal Tying Forceps
Purpose	To tie very fine suture material (e.g., 10/0 Polyglactin 9/0)
Size	11 cm (length)
Distinguishing Features	Fine 'buck tooth' like tips
Similar Instruments	MacPherson Tying Forceps

Forceps

Name	Capsule Forceps
Purpose	To grab the anterior lens capsule during extra-capsular cataract extraction
Size	11 cm (length)
Distinguishing Features	Cross action, wide handle
Similar Instruments	None

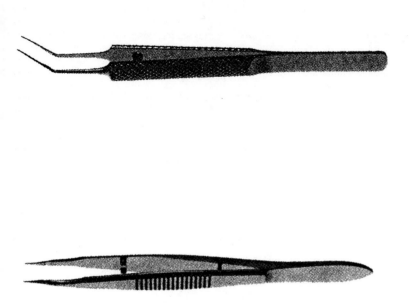

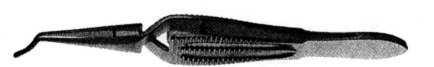

Hook

Name	Kirby Expressor Hook and Lens Loop
Purpose	Used during extra-capsular and intra-capsular lens removal The hook is used from the outside to put pressure on the lens and exteriorise it The loop is placed into the anterior chamber to help 'catch' the lens
Size	15 cm long
Distinguishing Features	It has a loop at one end and a blunt hook at the other
Similar Instruments	None have this combination

Speculum

Name	Williams Speculum
Purpose	To retract eyelids to allow access to eye ball
Size	8.5 cm long
Distinguishing Features	An adjustable screw at distal end to allow self retention
Similar Instruments	Clark and Lang Speculae

Speculum

Name	Barraquer Speculum
Purpose	To retract eye lids to allow access to the eye ball
Size	5 cm long
Distinguishing Features	Small fine speculum with no screw adjustment
Similar Instruments	Brown and Pierse Speculae

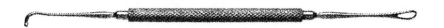

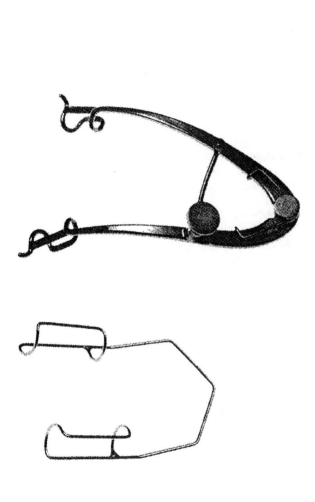

Dilator

Name	Nettleship Dilator
Purpose	To dilate narrow canals, eg, lacrimal duct
Size	11 cm
Distinguishing Features	It looks like a miniature javelin with longitudinal lines along the handle
Similar Instruments	Wilder Lacrimal Dilator (cross-hatching along the handle)

Needle Holders

Name	Castroviejo (Micro) Needle Holders
Purpose	Holding needles for suturing
Size	13 cm (length)
Distinguishing Features	Flat handles with no finger rings
Similar Instruments	Weiss, Troutman and Catford

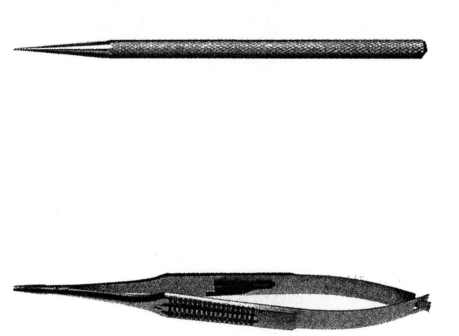

Dental Instruments

Common Features

All hand instruments should be held in a modified pen grip

Many hand instruments are superficially similar and need careful studying to recognise their differences

Extraction Forceps

Name   Extraction Forceps (small and large)

Purpose   Extraction of the multi-rooted teeth in the dog and cat

Size   15 cm long (small), 20 cm long (large)

Distinguishing Features Cup like cutting tips (similar to rongeurs)

Similar Instruments   Calculus Forceps

Dental Elevator

Name   Dental Elevator (chisel)

Purpose   To separate the attachment of the tooth root to the alveolar bone

Size   A variety of tip sizes to fit teeth of differing size and root diameter

Distinguishing Features Single ended instrument with relatively large hexagonal or octagonal handles

Periosteal Elevator

Name   Periosteal Elevator (double ended)

Purpose   To elevate the gingiva to expose bone during tooth extractions and oral surgery

Size   16 cm long

Distinguishing Features Angled, rounded tip

Similar Instruments   Dental Mixing Spatula, Dental Luxator

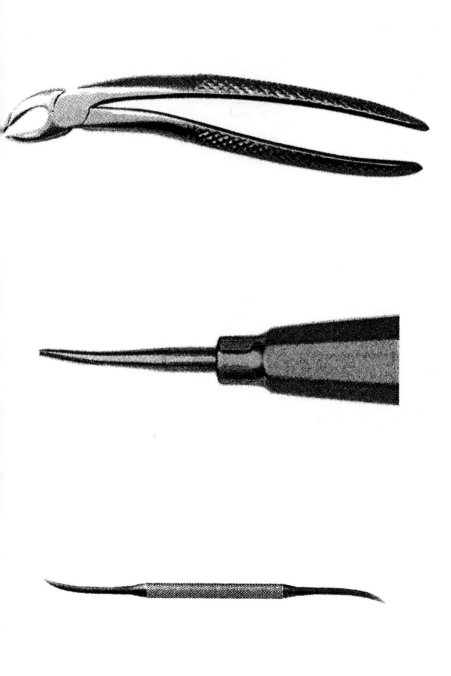

Subgingival Curette

Name	Subgingival Curette
	Universal: two cutting surfaces allowing either side to be used
	Dedicated: one cutting surface allowing one side only to be used
Purpose	To remove deposits of food, plaque and calculus from the subgingival area
Size	16 cm long
Distinguishing Features	The blade has a rounded tip and the back is curved
Similar Instruments	Supragingival scaler

Supragingival Scaler

Name	Supragingival Scaler
	Universal: two cutting surfaces allowing either side to be used
	Dedicated: one cutting surface allowing one side only to be used
Purpose	To remove deposits of food, plaque and calculus from the supragingival portion of the tooth surface
Size	16 cm long
Distinguishing Features	The blade is pointed and triangular in section
Similar Instruments	Subgingival curette

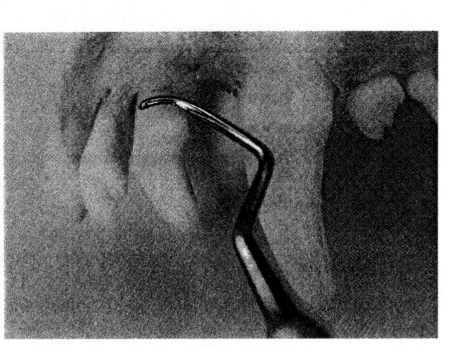

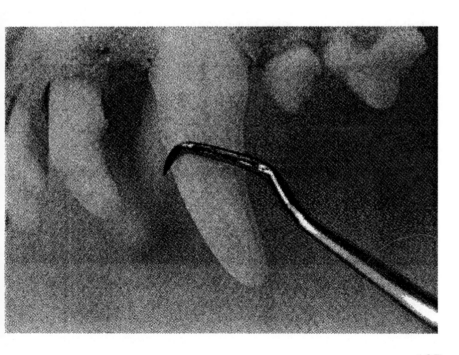

107

Dental Explorer

Name	Dental Explorer
Purpose	To explore the hard surface of teeth
Size	16 cm long
Distinguishing Features	Shepherd's hook type sharp tip for use on tooth surface only
Similar Instruments	Probe

Peridontal Probe

Name	Peridontal Probe
Purpose	To be inserted into the gingival sulcus next to a tooth to measure its depth or that of any peridontal pocket that is present
Size	16 cm long
Distinguishing Features	Blunt, rounded tip graduated to assist measurement of pocket depth
Similar Instruments	Explorer

Sharpening Stone

Name	Sharpening Stone
Purpose	Fine stone for sharpening peridontal instruments
Size	Various
Distinguishing Features	Made of stone
Similar Instruments	None

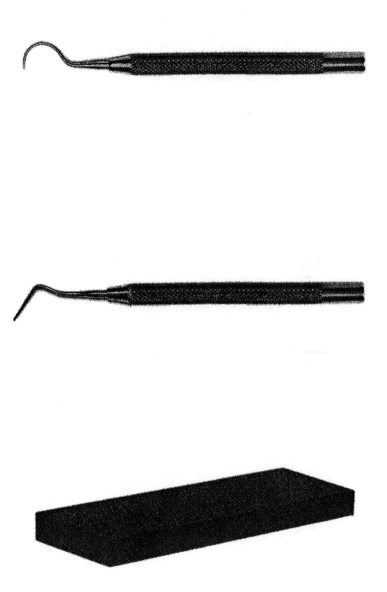

Miscellaneous Instruments

Cusco Vaginal Speculum

Name   Cusco Vaginal Speculum

Purpose   To retract tissue to expose other tissue

Size   Small, medium and large

Distinguishing Features   Duck bill shaped blades

Similar Instruments   Kilian (nasal speculum) for small/young animals

Hartmann Crocodile Forceps

Name   Hartmann Crocodile Forceps (plain)

Purpose   For aural and nasal use

Size   7 cm

Distinguishing Features   Crocodile type jaws at tips

Similar Instruments   Mattieus, swiss pattern

Rampley sponge holding forceps

Name   Rampley Sponge Holding Forceps

Purpose   Holding sponges or swabs for skin preparation prior
                          to surgery

Size   18 cm, 24 cm

Distinguishing Features   Flattened pear shaped ends

Similar Instruments   Foerster

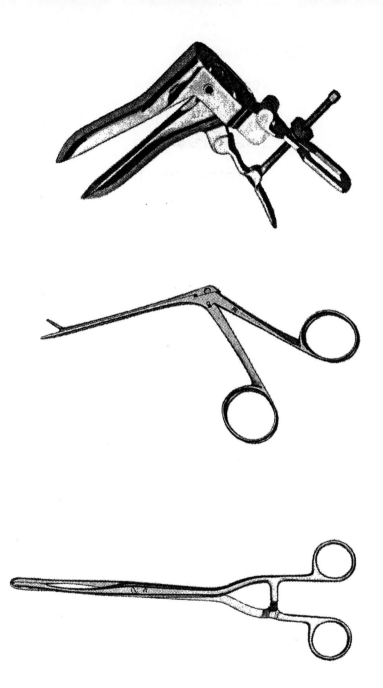

Cheatle Sterilising Forceps

Name	Cheatle Sterilising Forceps
Purpose	Sterile opening of packs by unscrubbed personnel
Size	27 cm and 29 cm
Distinguishing Features	Angled beak shaped tips
Similar Instrument	None

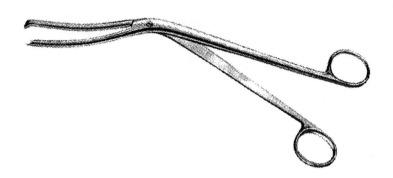

115

Lightning Source UK Ltd.
Milton Keynes UK
04 March 2010
150898UK00001B/25/A

9 780750 636131